Energizing Work

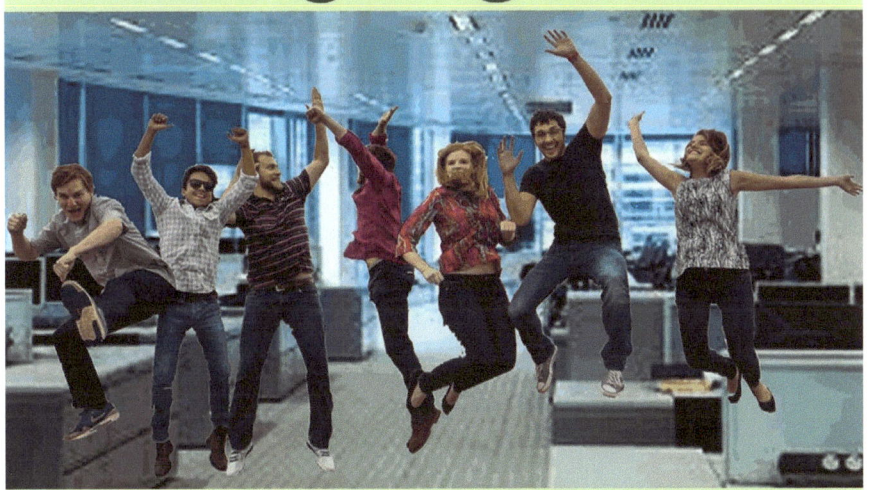

How work evolved to dominate life, and how to regain
balance & abundance!

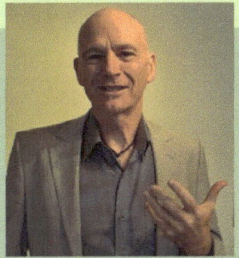

Phil "Philosofree" Cheney

Energizing Work

A reflection on work and its place in life.

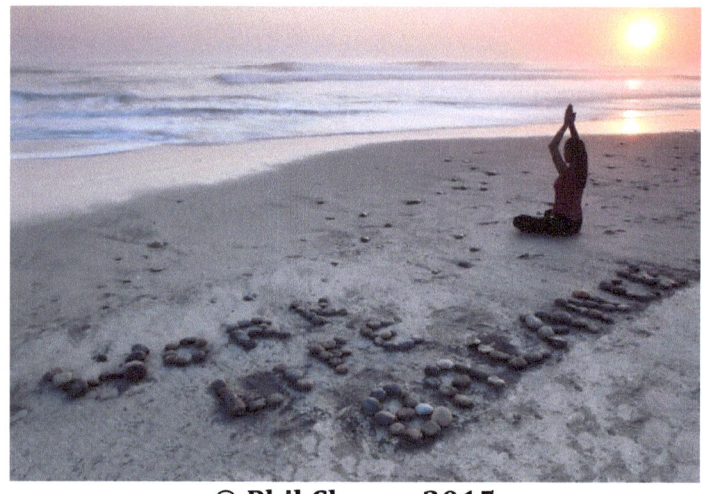

Contents

Preface

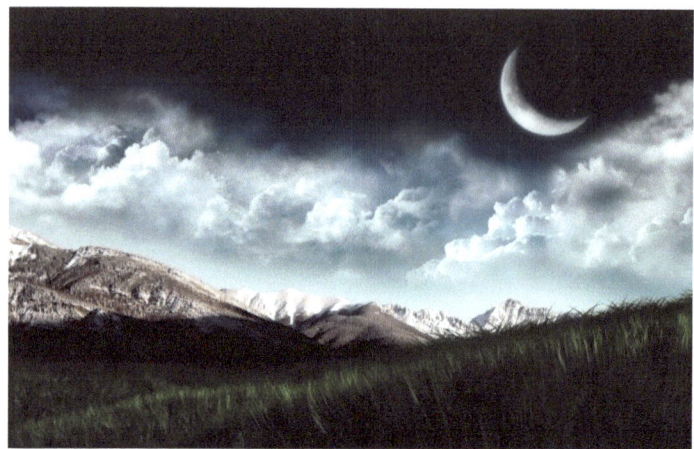

> "Success is neither magical nor mysterious.
> Success is the natural consequence of consistently
> applying the basic fundamentals."
>
> "Ideas can be life-changing. Sometimes all you
> need to open the door is just one more good idea."
>
> Jim Rohn

Jim Rohn was a good leader and an inspiring speaker, and I was fortunate enough to meet him when he was alive.
This book is about the energy that we all have access to that can entirely liberate how we see work, and how to apply the basic fundamentals in order to use our energies so that we can enjoy everything we do, both work and play.

For me, this is a life changing belief, and one that forms the core of my life and of this book.

Enjoy.
Phil 'Philosofree' Cheney
April 2015

Introduction

In our days people don't work anymore to make a living but they live for working. The average worker in the USA is now working one month more per year than 20 years ago. That is not counting travel time, which can add hours per day, and really should be taken into account as time hogging related to work.

However, having an engaging job and workplace *still trumps these factors* in fostering high overall well being in workers.
Those who were engaged in their work but took less than one week of vacation had 25% higher overall assessed well-being than actively disengaged employees, even those with six or more weeks of vacation.

What is well-being? Satisfaction. Enjoyment of each day. A feeling of purpose. Being healthily content. All of these flavors wrapped up in an ice-cream cone of happiness.

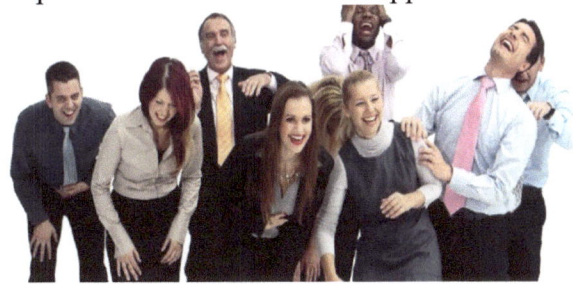

It seems like a fulfilling career influences our well-being as do other parts of our lives which are just as important. If you concentrate on work to the exclusion of (say) family, you may be happy in your dedication to making money, but a kick back occurs when you face your inner motives; why did you choose to do that in the first place? This is the big question, why do you put up with spending 40-60 hours each week doing work you may not want to be doing, when you can optimally be spending that same time doing what you love to do? Money? Your family obligations?

Hmm. Think about it. So many people today work long hours to pay for someone else to look after their children; cooking their meals, training them to exercise, ensuring that they eat properly, or for entertainment. All of these can be enjoyable, substituted with your own time. Oh you want flexibility and freedom? That makes sense. Engaged employees with a lot of flextime have 44 % higher well-being than actively disengaged employees with very little or no flextime.

Given that work is such an integral part of most western lives, what is it that you, the reader, want as a work/life balance? How do we energize work without stripping out health, relationships, hobbies, and indeed our own spirituality and sense of being?
True happiness lies in what you truly love.

What you love may be a certain person in your life or a passion that you can't get out of your head. True happiness envelopes you in a completely different world that shields you from the atrocities of our own perceptions. True happiness ascends us higher than we can ever imagine.

The issue is that many people genuinely believe that the person with the most toys wins. Then illness or age or divorce or any other aspect of life happens and toys become suddenly irrelevant.

This book provides a look at how to energize your work, and that implies satisfaction with the rest of your life and death.
Clarity, which is the focus of the Advantace brand, helps us to differentiate between the things we do, and the things we are.
Initially we will look at how what we do has changed and continues to change over time. Then we will consider: Why we do what we do? What drives us to want more, to do more, to consume more?

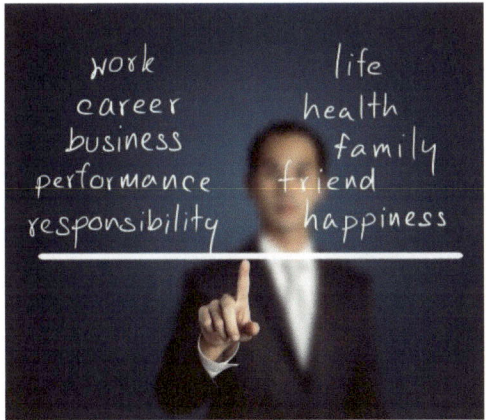

Then the issue of being is considered. What constitutes being? Can we even differentiate being as opposed to doing?

Do you identify 'being' with 'being lazy'? How can we distinguish between what little it takes to survive, and what we are afraid of if we consider such a low bar on survival? Why do we work for decades in order to retire and what does retirement mean?

The things we do

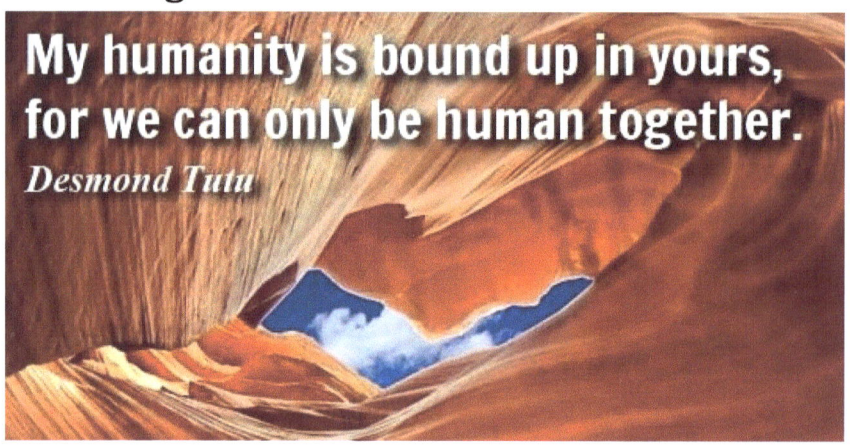

My humanity is bound up in yours,
for we can only be human together.

Desmond Tutu

> Some people would claim that things like love, joy and beauty belong to a different category from science and can't be described in scientific terms, but I think they can now be explained by the theory of evolution.
>
> Stephen Hawking

What we do now

I don't work 9-5 anymore. I used to for decades, and although sometimes it was in employment I loved, it also included work I would rather not have been doing.

Then I chose to work at what I want to do, to make a break from the 'rat race' and I am now happier than ever before. I spend about the same number of hours **doing** non-play activities as I used to but it is from choice. Also the hours I allocate to generating income are enjoyable. Sometimes I do stone masonry, because I love it. Sometimes I write because I love it. Sometimes I do housework….

Now hang on, you say, surely you don't love ***housework***?
Well that is a good question. Let me ask you this, think of an activity that required discipline and repetition, digging the garden,

exercising at a gym, learning a musical instrument. Thought of one? Good. I suggest that the attitude towards that activity is what determined your memory of it being wonderful or a drudge. Which one was the one you chose? Now choose one that was the opposite type, if you chose a negative activity, choose a positive, or vice versa.

What was the difference? Both had repetition, like say doing dishes, both had discipline, in that you had to choose over something that may have been less effort. The old concept of "chop wood, carry water" as a way of achieving bliss has merit. Being entertained by someone else's life hasn't the power to revolutionize your own.

So yes, I do love housework when my desire to do it is positive; when my intention is to have a clean house, to enjoy and appreciate a meal cooked by my own hands, or to enjoy hanging up clothes because I want time in the fresh air. Often our intentions towards activities which are labelled 'work' are the same. We have generations of perception embedded in our genes, much of it post-industrial age angst against being treated like machines. But we each have the capability of turning that around. We can choose each day, to act, to **DO**, as we wish.

You think this is not possible, that you would die from lack of food or shelter? The basics are dealt with in a later chapter, but in the western world the basic requirements are often overshadowed with other people's expectations. We are not working for food, most of the time, but for approval, for a better education for the kids, because our mother-in-law has higher expectations on the sort of house we should live in, etc.

How can we break out of this cycle of other-people-make-work-a-chore?
Firstly, let us look at the history of work, how it has changed, and how that change is accelerating.

A short history of work as a societal perception.

Jump back a bit in time, say 10,000 years, and consider how people lived.

"*Philosophers, mystics from many wisdom traditions, psychologists, and neuroscientists have all delved into this most fascinating question: how has human consciousness evolved from the time we lived in caves to who we are today?*" (Frederic Laloux).

Does it seem that things appear to have changed? Yes. Society has a strong influence on individual activity.

Let's see how the way of doing things has evolved in the history of humanity. The stages of community are explained as they appear in the book "Reinventing Organizations" by Frederick Laloux.

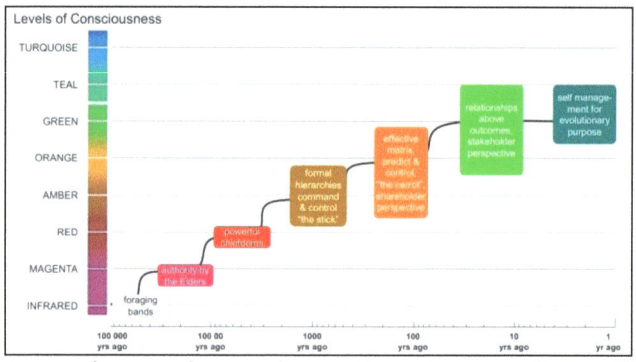

The picture above shows how the stages of consciousness developed through time according to Frederick Laloux.

"*There is nothing inherently "better" about being at a higher level of development, just as an adolescent is not "better" than a toddler. However, the fact remains that an adolescent is able to do more, because he or she can think in more sophisticated ways than a toddler. Any level of development is okay; the question is whether that level of development is a good fit for the task at hand.*" (Nick Petrie). That quote shows us that in our current state of mind we are not better than our ancestors. In fact without them we wouldn't be in that place at all.

Let's do a quick tour through work and play during the last 100,000 years of human consciousness, by considering important stages of cultural impact, named as colors. While humanity needed 50,000 years to change from Infrared to Magenta, you can see in the following graph how human awareness/consciousness is accelerating in the last 100 years.

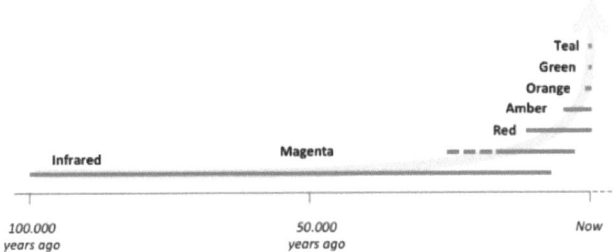

So, what stage of human consciousness does every color represent?

Development of Consciousness

The color **Infrared** indicates the earliest development stage. In that time, small family kinships lived together as gatherers and hunters. There was no division of work yet, except that the women were usually responsible to raise the group's children. People in that stage had no fully developed ego yet and did not know about hierarchies or leadership. Fostering was then what we now would describe as working. It was necessary to get food to survive.

The Infrared stage lasted tens of thousands of years until something changed.

Magenta-Magic

The small family clans of a few dozen people opened up and humans started to live in bigger groups or tribes that consisted of a few hundred people. Humans started to see themselves more separate from other individuals. This stage of consciousness was labeled as magical by some authors as cause and effect were still hardly understood and the world seemed to be full of spiritual things to explain the unexplainable. Work was still not divided in the **Magenta-Magic** stage.

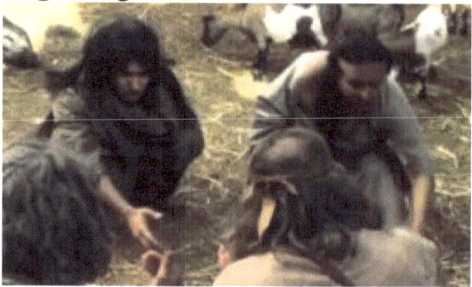

Ancient civilizations contained magenta elements, too. The following quotes by the ancient Greek philosopher Heraclitus seem relevant until today:

Most people do not understand the things they experience, nor do they know what they have learned; but they seem to themselves to have done so.

Those who do not understand, when they hear are like the deaf.

What can we take from that? Often, people see events and their direct cause in a very small point of view missing the bigger picture. If eating a chocolate cake makes you feel happy, that's actually your personal opinion. People tend to mix up their own opinions with true understanding of the world.

Those who do not understand, when they hear are like the deaf.

A similar meaning can be found in the above quote: People read or hear something and only look at the meaning of the words, but they miss to look behind them and find out their true value.

What sense or thought do they have? They follow the popular singers, and they take the crowd as their teacher.

Yes, people take opinions of others and make them to their own without even question them. They don't think by themselves and are swept down the river.

Red-Leadership

With the **Red stage** humanity reached a breakthrough point as division of work developed. For the first time, humans realized the inevitable reality of death. With that implementation the world becomes a scary place and you had to be strong to satisfy your needs. With strength also came submission, the less powerful submitted themselves to stronger ones in the hope of getting their needs met by said arrangement. In other words, if you work for somebody more powerful, that person gets his work done and might pay back for that convenience. Simple hierarchy developed that empowered the tougher ones to rule above the weaker who were trapped in dependency. Violence is still a way to express your needs while one is still quite unaware of other people's feelings.

You might say that Red people had only manual labor at that time, but consider this, that when you spend your work days typically in an office or in transit, and then intentionally go to a gym to do what came naturally back then, was the exercise a problem, or is it attitude? Consider how you worry about not being healthy because you don't work out enough. Go figure…

Amber-Conformist

When humans started to become farmers, the **Amber-Conformist** stage was reached. It was a giant step forward but it brought with it new types of control like states, civilizations, institutions, bureaucracy and religion. The former impulsive Red behavior gave way to self-discipline and self-control. Only if you save seeds from this year's harvest, you will have food next year, too. As you can see, in the Amber stage people were able to divide between past, present and future. Cause and effect were understood. If I do this today, it will have that influence on tomorrow. Complex and stable hierarchies formed, the nutritious food provided by farmers made it possible that others could focus on different professions. The shift to agriculture enabled the development of countries and civilizations in the first place.

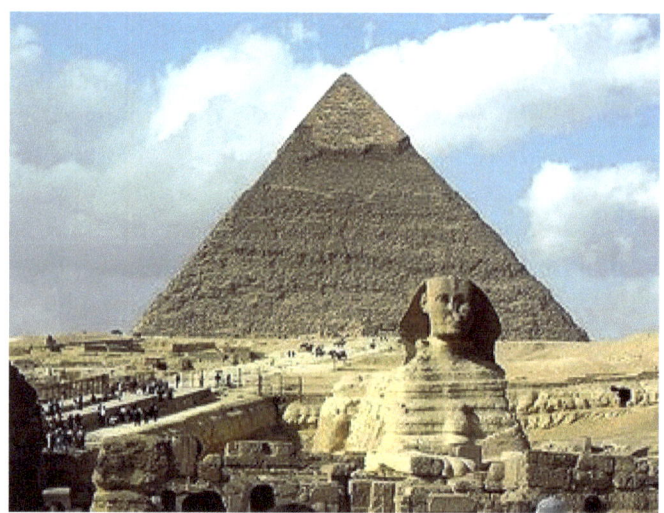

With civilizations came simple ideas of morality based on one idea what is right and what is wrong. People started to develop empathy and care for each other, but limited to groups. If you behave in the accepted way, you will be rewarded, if you do wrong, you will be punished and maybe even banned from the group.

The command and control push from the top of the hierarchy down to the bottom and there is no movement or development in Conformist-Amber: The future is only a repetition of the past; there is no learning or change.

Developmental psychologists believe, that the majority of today's adults acts as Conformist-Amber and a lot of institutions are still organized that way, for example the army, the Catholic Church and most government agencies.

Orange-Achievement

The **Orange-Achievement** stage was reached when the Industrial Revolution turned people's way of living upside down. The world-view changed from "we are the center of the universe" to "we are only a small part in a huge and complex system". Scientists started to investigate the laws of nature, companies developed. Achievement is everything now, developing something new gives power and success.

The worldview is not black and white anymore, but it's very materialistic. What is not visible is not real. Obviously, spirituality is having a hard time. To be orange means to live in the future, more is better. The more we achieve or own, the happier we will be, but the current state is never happy enough. The Orange stage gave humanity so much; our whole lifestyle is based on that, no smartphone without the invention of the steam engine. When will we figure that more is not always better, that we cannot buy happiness?

I recommend having a look at this blog post: https://www.blinkist.com/page19/coal-mines-cubicles-way-work-broken-fix

Here is an orange view of the world, from that post:
"Industrial revolution work policies were no cup of English breakfast. Work in factory textile mills and coal mines was typified by:

- A strict command hierarchy in which decisions were made at the top and implemented at the bottom.
- A large army of uneducated minions who performed mindless work like swinging a pickaxe or operating a mechanical loom, with middle managers barking orders at them.

- A thoroughly unpleasant organizational culture for all involved, except maybe the cigar-smoking, top hat-wearing, monocle-wiping owner at the top of the hierarchy.

Although things have changed for the more humane since then, if reading the above gave you an unsettling prickle of familiarity, you wouldn't be alone. This system of management, called *command and control*, is still widely used today.

Command and control might be "historically proven," but it only makes sense if the person running the show is a complete genius, and the employees, mental midgets incapable of independent thought. These days though, organizations tend not to be this stratified: smart, educated people can be found at all levels of a company, and as you've probably already realized if you've ever held a job, that someone holds a senior position doesn't always indicate smarts.

So what do you think happens when you try to force people of equal intelligence into a strict hierarchy as in the command and control system?

71% of people wind up hating their jobs, that's what."

Like many of the old technologies, orange management is still alive and kicking. Unfortunately it kicks and hurts. Something had to change..

Green-Equality

This stage started in the end of the 19th century in industrial countries. It learned from Orange's mistakes and tried to work on them. Green leaders want to burst through the walls of hierarchy and separation and bring equality. That leads to disentanglement of old structures like patriarchy, social classes and institutional religion. It was the time of the battle for women's rights and against slavery and apartheid. These liberation movements are still going on all over the world, because equality is not yet reached. Green means empowerment, harmony, fairness, community and consensus. In Orange, community was lost, Green rediscovers it. In Green there is no egoism anymore, it's not about what's best for me but what's right for everybody.

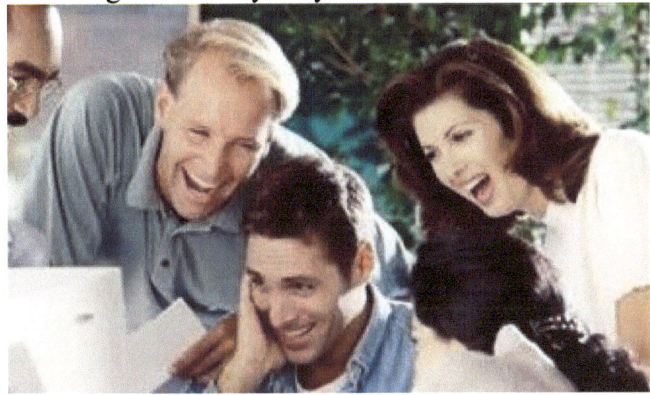

Evolutionary-Teal

Evolutionary-Teal is the next step, some have already taken the leap, some are not there yet, but it is happening now. Teal is about inner rightness, where we question our behaviors and try to live up to the goal to discover our true selves. We disengage from our fears, as we stop to worry about the future; we reach more freedom in decision making. We stop to plan ahead and instead try to react on current situations. A good life is no longer defined by wealth or success. We consider us as a part of some bigger energy that connects us with life and nature itself.

Survival is no longer sufficient. Our evolution now requires us to develop spiritually - to become emotionally aware and make responsible choices. It requires us to align ourselves with the values of the soul - harmony, cooperation, sharing, and reverence for life.

Gary Zukav

Advantace offers executive coaching, incorporating life coaching and clarity coaching.

Clarity coaching follows the Evolutionary-Teal objectives of the emerging organization;

- Treating life as a journey of unfolding instead of pre-planned goals and routes
- Internal yardsticks to measure growth towards your true nature and your calling
- A life well-lived breeds success, profit etc., not vice versa
- Focus on strengths, not on failures and what's wrong
- There are no mistakes, only opportunities to learn

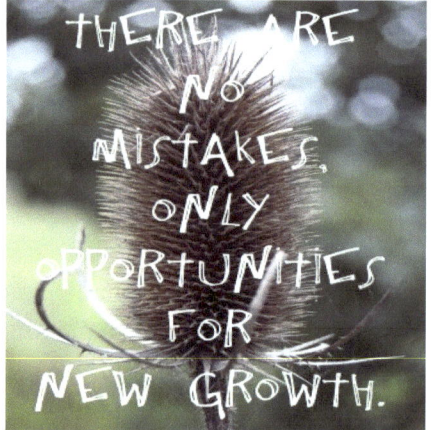

- Wisdom valued beyond rationality
- 'Both-and' thinking instead of dualistic 'either-or'
- Integrating mind-body-soul
- Being true to yourself
- Striving for wholeness with Self, others, life, nature

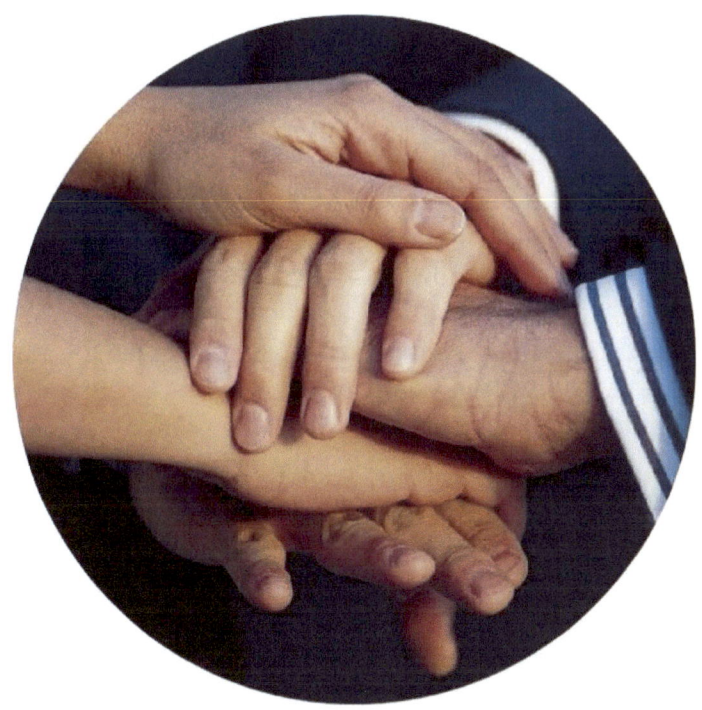

This approach is not just a theory; it is the working framework for many successful organizations today, and it is revolutionizing the lives of the participants.

Retirement

How is it that many people still hold on to the concept of retirement meaning to stop work? Surely that definition ignores the opening concepts of loving what we do. If we love what we do, why would we want to stop?

On the other hand, if we no longer have to earn, because our career has generated financial stability, retirement opens up new possibilities of defining work. Think of the retirees who have gone back to university to get a degree in a subject they love, who have opened a new business. My mother started wood carving at age 75 and had completed over 300 major pieces before her death. It was not work for her.

What are you working for? It should not be to stop working, because that means you don't love what you are working at. Better to find what you love and convert now, and that includes loving the social and home repetitions, the overall experience of joy that comes from doing something that you have chosen to do, and that you want to do well.

Thich Nat Hahn is a great exponent of being in the here and now, enjoying what is set before you, and choosing to do it well.

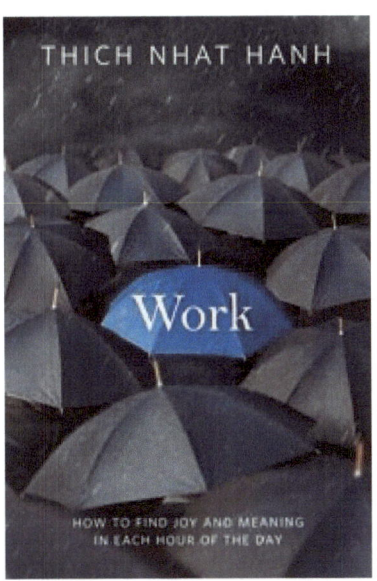

You can find his book "Work" on Amazon or bookstores.

Thich Nhat Hanh adapts ancient Buddhist practices to modern life and helps readers make fulfilling choices about livelihood and ethical work. Full of life-coaching advice, tips for finding happiness and changing habits Work suggest new mindful models of leadership and encourages us to carefully examine our everyday choices, so we can contribute to a work environment free from stress and tension, regardless of the circumstance.

The things we do can be changed, by looking at who we are.

The things we are

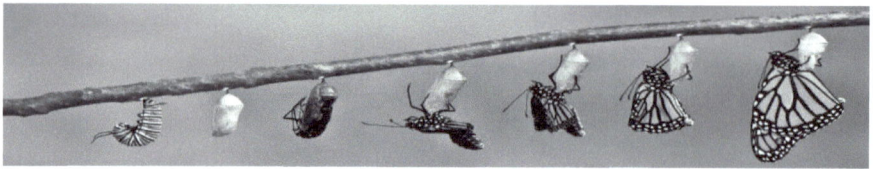

> The most exciting breakthroughs of the twenty-first century will not occur because of technology, but because of an expanding concept of what it means to be human.
>
> John Naisbitt

Firstly, let's consider how you see yourself and how your relationship towards yourself is.

Self-Confident

As soon as you trust yourself, you will know how to live
(Johann Wolfgang von Goethe - Faust: First Part)

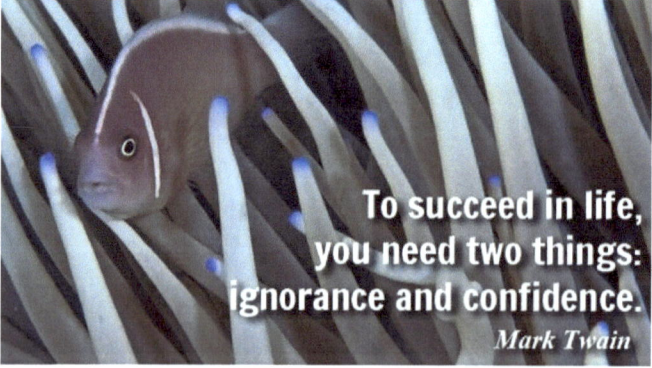

To succeed in life, you need two things: ignorance and confidence.
Mark Twain

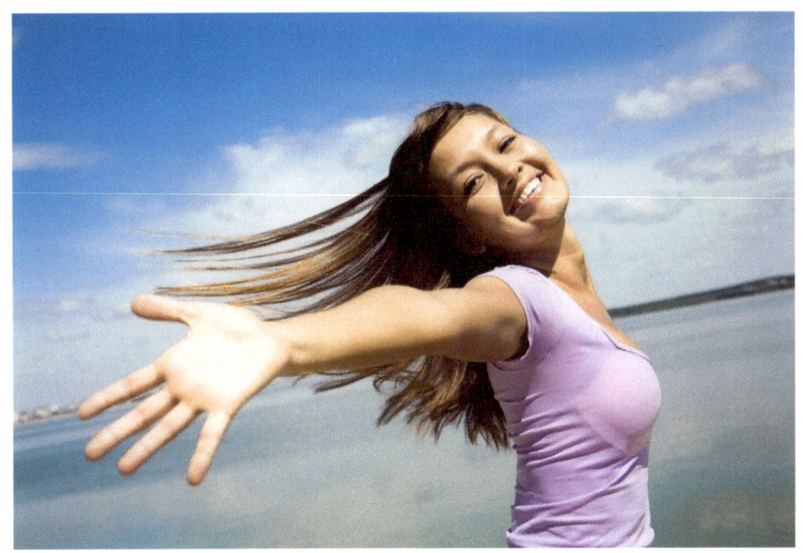

To be self-confident is a good start. Believing in yourself is so important, however if you are a woman, then this is going to be more difficult than for a man.

That's because media conveys images of "the perfect woman" which are impossible for most of them to achieve. It may be how to appear, what to wear or how to behave – women still face many more regulations by their environment than men. It's part of a patriarchal ideology that's still hard to overcome.

If you see yourself as a woman strong and confident about yourself you will be less open to this false image. Especially in male-dominated professions you may still face everyday sexism which can affect your self-esteem. Don't let it come that far. Strong self-confidence and supporting people at your side will help you with that.

When you're different, sometime you don't see the millions of people who accept you for what you are. All you notice is the person who doesn't.
(Jodi Picoult - Change of Heart)

If you take time off from work, do you feel lost and then look around for something to do in order to settle yourself? Is this because you identify 'being inactive' with 'being lazy'?

Do you feel guilty when you call in sick or you leave work earlier than usual because you don't feel good? That leads us straight to the next point.

Healthy

How healthy are you?
Do you have a healthy and well-balanced diet?
Do you exercise regularly?
Do you drink enough water every day?

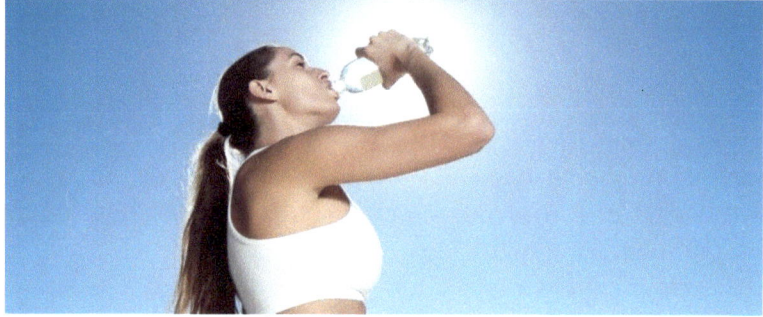

Do you get enough sleep every night?

If you feel less motivated and energized in the day, maybe you don't take care enough of your body. Our body is our temple, and we need to preserve it to have a healthy life.

It is shocking to know that over 65% of all Westerners are either obese or overweight. That's insane!

Think of your body as your physical vehicle to take you through life. If you repeatedly abuse the vehicle with unhealthy food and bad habits, it will wear out quickly.

Maybe you look fine from the outside, while on the insight, your arteries are getting clogged up with cholesterol and arterial plaque. That's not a pretty sight!
Today, your vital organs (kidney, heart, lungs, gall bladder, liver, stomach, intestines, etc.) may be working well, but they may not tomorrow.

Don't take your good health today for granted.

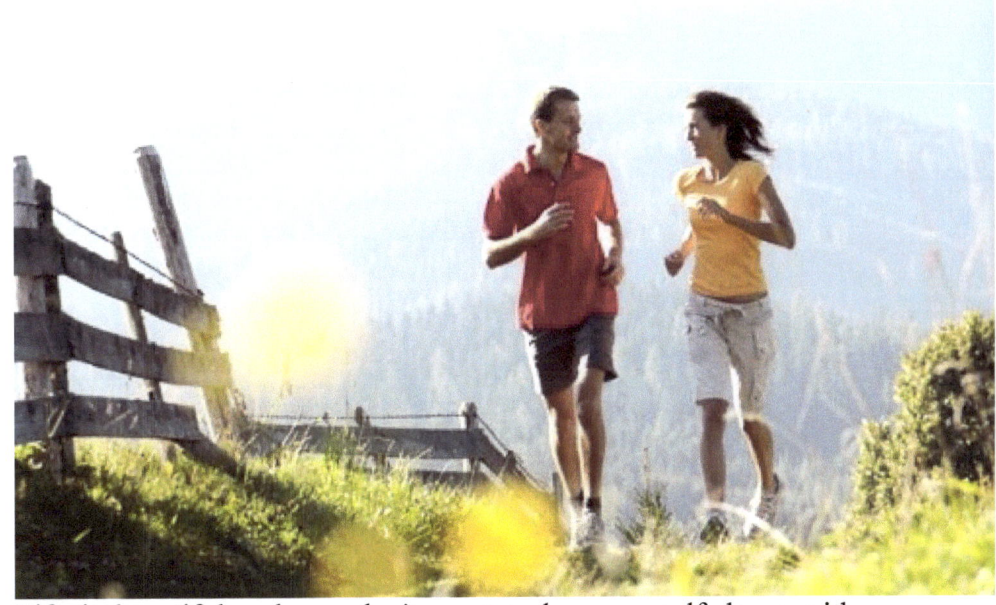

Life is beautiful and you don't want to bog yourself down with unnecessary health problems.

Of course, we cannot protect ourselves from any kind of disease, sometimes fate or our genetics or both betray us, but a healthy lifestyle can prevent us from getting sick.

Good health isn't just about healthy eating and exercise – it also includes having a positive mental health, self-image and a healthy lifestyle.

Independent

Why do you rely on others in order to survive?
Who do you assess as critical, and why?

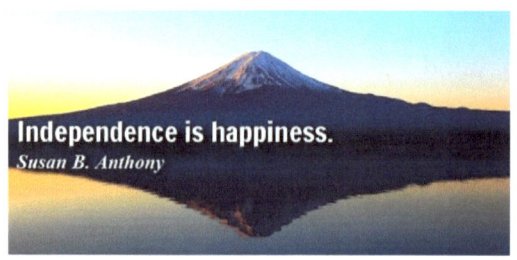

Independence is happiness.
Susan B. Anthony

These questions lead to an understanding of what independence actually is. Of course we need relationships, but when you find that you are not being authentic in relationships in any part of your life, at that point you are also being dishonest with yourself.

It is worth considering how comfortable are you with being quiet with yourself, just in alone time. We really are different in our tolerance levels for alone time, but being alone, without any media input, is a good test of independence:

Can you even do it, and if so for how long?

Try this simple test, the 10 minute test. Find a place where you are on your own, without any distractions, no mobile, no phone, no TV or devices, no sound, no interruptions, and just listen to your own breathing. Just 10 minutes.

Don't take this book or any other, just sit comfortably and listen. Listen to who you are as a body. You exist. Without work, or other people, you exist. If your mind wanders when doing the 10 minute test, consider this question to bring back your focus. "How much do I love my own company?"

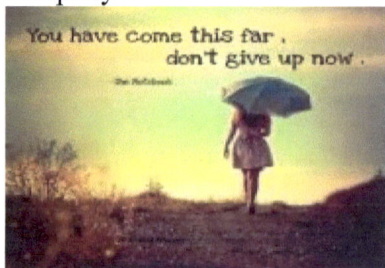

You have come this far, don't give up now.

While there is no "right" or "wrong" in this, it is my belief that being able to spend time alone and enjoy your own company is a sign of mental health.

It reflects a strong inner core and a good sense of self-esteem. And if we are happy and comfortable with whom we are, we are less dependent of other people's company.

If you do not experience a strong sense of self, a solid core inside (**a belief that you can maneuver through life effectively**), you can easily feel as if you are on the ocean, in an inadequate boat, in the midst of a storm. You *need* reassurance and the comfort of others to help provide a sense of grounding and well-being.

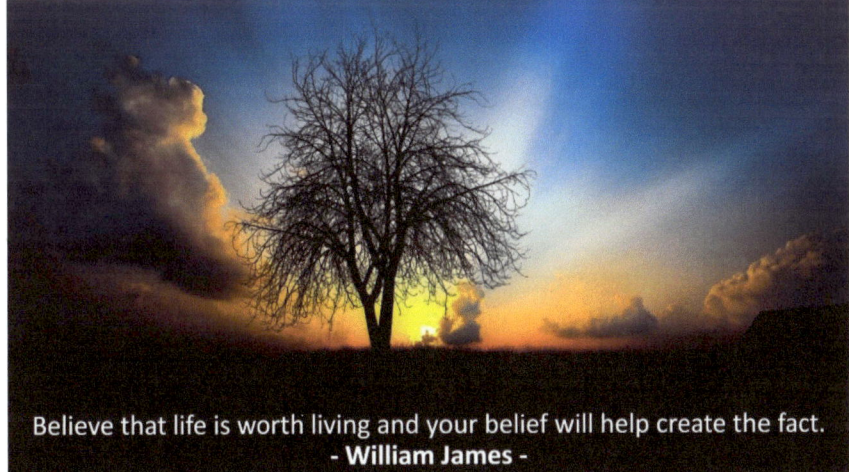

Believe that life is worth living and your belief will help create the fact.
- William James -

While most of us want occasional reassurance, life is ever so much more enjoyable when you know how to self-soothe and provide your own sense of comfort.

Self-soothing

Self-soothing involves being able to talk with yourself in a manner that is reassuring and calming.

An example might be: "I know I am feeling scared right now, but I'll be okay. I've experienced this feeling before and I survived it. I think I'll take a warm bath and listen to beautiful music."

If you feel "empty" inside, it is difficult to be alone, maybe even excruciating. Self-soothing can be a great tool to begin to deal with these feelings.

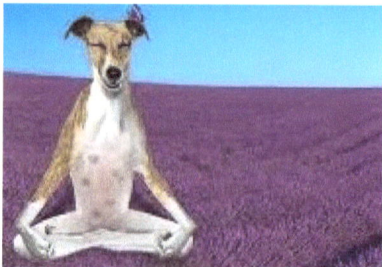

I love this analogy: If you came upon a child who was hiding in a closet afraid, would you say: "Come on out of there you little brat?" Or would you soothe the child?
Soothe yourself when you are fearful.

"If you're lonely when you're alone, you're in bad company."
(Jean-Paul Sartre)

If we don't love ourselves then what does that say about our being?

How can we distinguish between what little it takes to survive, and what we are afraid of if we consider such a low bar on survival?

Why do we work for decades in order to retire and what does retirement mean? (See the later chapter on Retirement)

Maybe we are indeed prisoners of a reduced understanding of the world. There is a simple story which can proof that:
How many brains does a human being have?

One, you might answer, but actually, there are three. The one in the head (we all know that), a small one in our heart and another one in the gut. The last ones where already discovered in the 1860s and then, scientists just forgot about them. They were rediscovered more than 130 years later by American neuroscientist Michael Gerson.

How could that even happen? One reason could be that the idea of three autonomous brains sharing the work does simply not feed the hierarchical worldview. There must be one boss or leader, that's how we saw the world for a long time.

Think about it: Is it really a coincidence that the two other brains were rediscovered in the same time as the Internet started to dominate our lives? The Internet revolutionized our world view and suddenly a shared intelligence and leadership seemed possible.

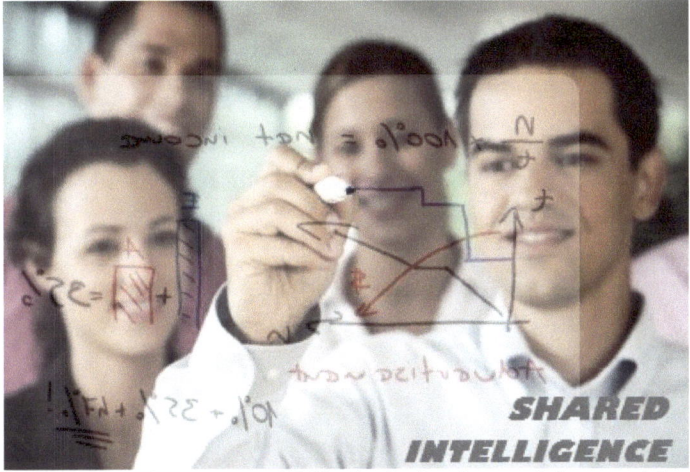

It is amazing that humans still limit their view of the world to what they are told, rather than to their experience. They believe everything without questioning it or trying to find more information on their own.

In my book "**Energizing Love**" the whole concept of a new view of shared intelligence, using genetic memory from prior generations, in the form of holographic inference patterns, is described. It has been known for a long time, but like looking at the other "brains" we have, modern western thinking has been blind to see.

Are you still under the spell of considering that being, spiritually, is akin to vegging out, to being lazy, to not being turned on? Once that concept is let go, you can discover other forms of being that will indeed energize your work, and your life. But how do you balance the two?

Balancing doing and being

The 1982 novel "Deadeye Dick" by the popular author Kurt Vonnegut mentioned the following piece of graffiti:

"To be is to do"– Socrates
"To do is to be"– Jean Paul Sartre
"Do be do be do"– Frank Sinatra

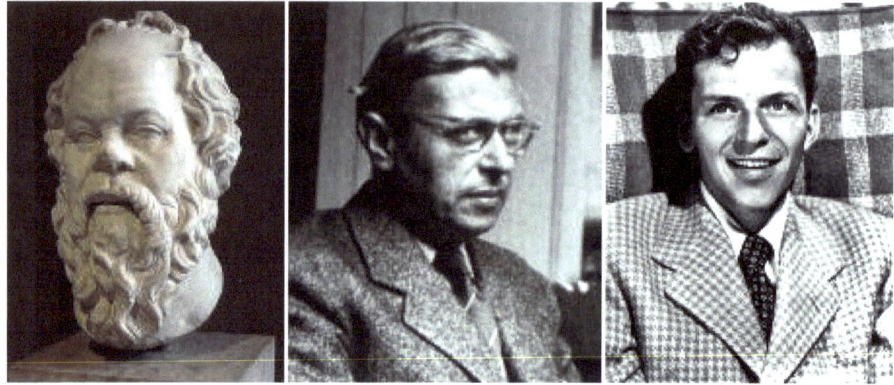

Socrates   **J. P. Sartre**   **Frank Sinatra**

Being, and being comfortable with it, is a great determinant of how we observe our doing. If you are doing in order to not face your emotions, you are probably not happy or peaceful.

> Fear is the cheapest room in the house. I would like to see you living in better conditions.
>
> Hafiz

Fear can exist in the broad light of the day but it takes it's strenght from the darkness. In that shabby, run-down room where fear rules, there is no light and it is filled with loud distractions that drowns the voice of our heart.

The radio or TV is always on, we never turn off the phone, and we try everything to cover that voice in us because we're afraid of what it says.

People can have everything and still live in a constant place of fear – and is that really a fulfilled live then?

Fear makes us worry about the future and therefore try to control the uncontrollable. The future becomes our enemy. Fear makes us numb and unable to enjoy what we have, because we always worry that we will lose it again.

But life offers us so much that we should move into a more expensive room and leave fear behind. Needless to say, life is not always fun and easy, there are scary and sad times, too, but they are part of the whole thing.

When we live in fear, permanently, we deprive ourselves of the possibility to truly live.

One way to visualize doing and being is to consider a porpoise. When it is in its world, it is part of the ocean, and is being.

When it leaps out of the water, it is a joyous celebration of existence; it is creative and fun doing.

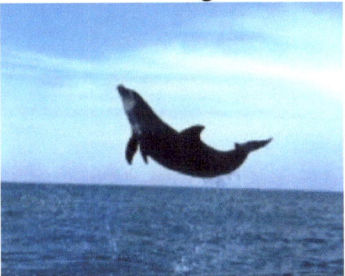

That is the optimum for us humans also. If we can emulate a porpoise, we will recognize that we are part of the human experience, that all of us are connected and part of the ocean of human existence. We just are, and are acceptable in that state.

Then once we feel and understand our worthiness, our belonging, to the ocean, we can jump out of our being and celebrate! If work and play are mixed in this way they can be a joyous and wonderful event, doing stuff that we love, not forced into anything. This is what Laloux's work teaches us, that when we come from a place of being accepted and loved, life is abundant and our physical doing can be an inspired and purposeful creation.

The following points may assist you to determine this:

Develop a vision

With a vision, you can be doing the most boring work and yet feel stimulated and satisfied, knowing that you are supporting a cause and a direction that you firmly believe in. For example, you may have a vision of becoming a racing driver, and to achieve that you work in the pits on menial work in order to get to understand the career, and to link with connections towards your goal.

Set a challenge

Challenges are seen as part and parcel of any job. Seek to innovate, test out new ideas and break away from the conventional way of doing things.

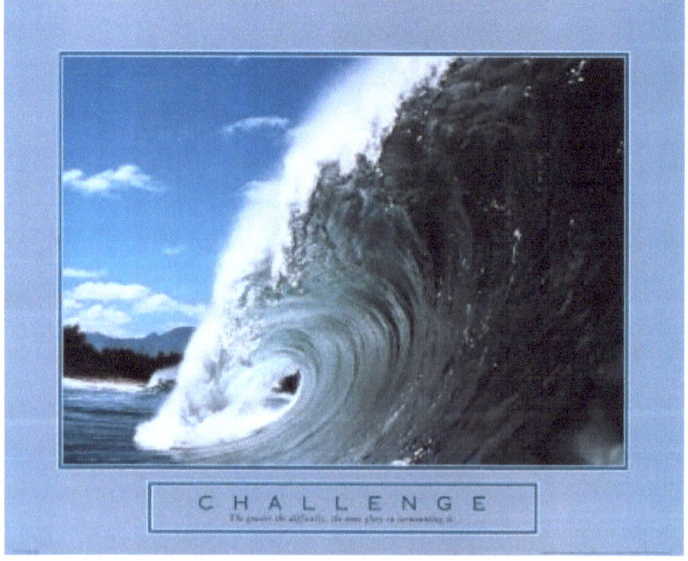

Be open-minded

Everyone needs a chance to stretch themselves to the limit. Fully motivated people have been described as those who feel they are the best at what they do, and can achieve whatever they imagine. To do so, be open to ideas from everyone who crosses your path. They, in turn, may provide new ideas, propose solutions to improve your life and, at the same time, you will be encouraged and rewarded with their help. That is what cooperation and a positive attitude allows.

Be participative

Be energetic, positive and always ready to get your hands dirty. We all admire those who lead by example. Develop confidence and trust in yourself by walking the talk. Go a step further to show others how to live, and you will learn more.

Enjoy your work.

If you are passionate about your work, very often you will be have a sense of fun in your work attitude. You will happily break rules to get things done. You will treat your work as play and truly enjoy what you are doing. You will be an asset in an organization and your biggest accomplishment will be to authentically enjoying what you create.

The vision and charisma you emit also unites all the others in your workplace to strive for peak performance and create the synergy essential for success.

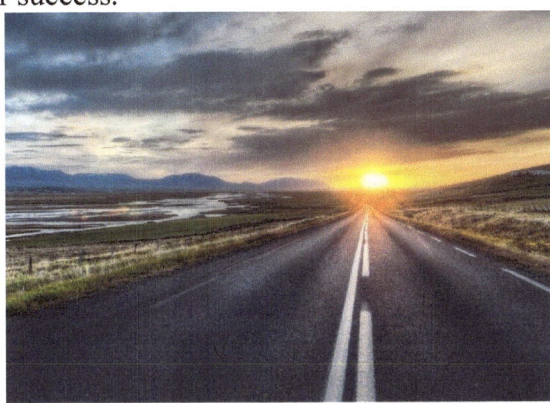

Once you have identified your motivation, you should ask yourself **"Where does my motivation arise from?"** Carrot and stick are two different approaches to motivating yourself. Do you apply a formal rule and apply guilt in your life and work, or do you use passion and emotions to motivate yourself?

In my book "Energizing Love" I propose that all creativity comes from intentional energy which is universal and takes the form of love. I will not go into that premise now, but simply ask you to consider where you feel most at ease in your life. I am asking for the feeling state of peace and purpose, not the space where you are blanked out like a couch potato.

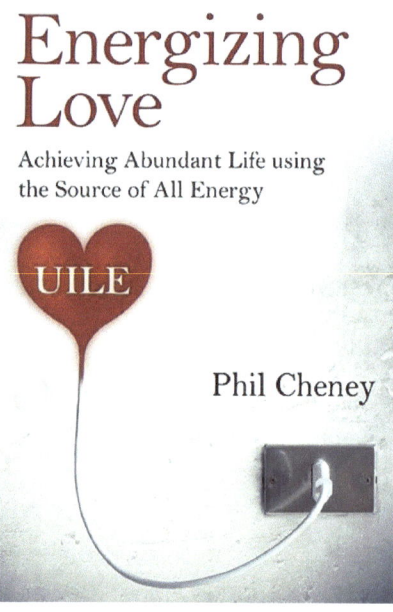

While there are many theories about motivation, it is, at its most basic, what prompts us to move towards a goal. These cues can be biological or psychological, conscious or unconscious. The mix can be complex and hard to understand.

If you find that what you're actually inclined to do and what you'd like to be inclined to do differ, then you have some decisions to make about whether to follow the course of least resistance or try to manipulate your motivation in some way – by changing your routines or reminding yourself of what you have to lose by not making an effort. The choice should have a lot to do with matters of value – whether the thing you need to push yourself to do is valuable in itself or will serve a valuable goal.

The distinction between intrinsic and extrinsic motivation could be a useful aid. The former refers to all the things you do for their own sake, and the latter to those you do as a means to an end. Work, for instance, can span the whole spectrum: from an intrinsic source of satisfaction to a necessary means towards the outcomes of earning a living or gaining social standing.

You've probably heard the saying 'true motivation comes from within' – which can be a bit of a cliché – but like many clichés there is a ring of truth about them.

I realized this when some years ago when I attended a seminar by a very well-known speaker (I don't want to say who) where I was absolutely mesmerized by their rhetoric and after a couple of hours left fired up and inspired to make some drastic changes to my life.

Unfortunately – the fire quickly disappeared – probably within a week and I quickly forgot all about it. I wasn't even really aware what had happened until a couple of months later. But then I came across this quote by Stephen Covey and it explained exactly what the problem is.

"Motivation is a fire from within. If someone else tries to light that fire under you, chances are it will burn very briefly."
Stephen R. Covey

Talk about a light bulb moment. Of course the speech hadn't made any real impact on me. The enthusiasm I had felt on the original day was all about him and his success and although I was impressed – that's all I was – impressed by his achievements. I kidded myself. I didn't actually think about how they related to me and how I really would make the changes I wanted. The motivation just wasn't there.

Foolishly I'd assumed that I could get someone else to motivate me. I'm not alone in this. I often get people asking me – can I help motivate them. The short answer is: I can't.

Maslow's Hierarchy of Needs

One of the main theories relating to motivation is **Maslow's Hierarchy of Needs**. Humans have needs.

A need is a lack of something – something we want. This produces the drive and desire which motivates us to satisfy that need. Satisfying this need, or getting the thing we want or lack is the goal. Maslow's hierarchy of needs is a theory in psychology proposed by the American psychologist Abraham Maslow in his 1943 paper "A Theory of Human Motivation". This is a theory of psychological health predicated on fulfilling innate human needs in priority, culminating in self-actualization.

Maslow believes that every human has five needs in the following order of importance

Physiological Needs represent the very basic needs of humanity: Without satisfying the needs for food, water and sleep we would die, the need to reproduce retains the human race from extinction.

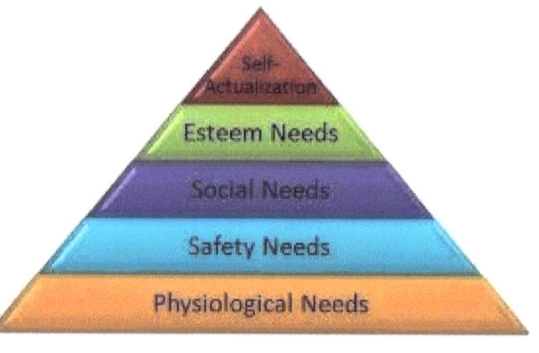

The need to work also belongs in the first category, because working ensures our survival.

Safety Needs
People have the need for a shelter and for feeling safe and protected. That means not only that we need to have a house or a

safe place, but the need for safety is also part of the reason why religions and science exist. Humans feel the urge to explain every phenomenon and they are afraid of the unknown.

Social Needs
This is the need to be part of a group and to be accepted by others. Without friends, a partner, a family, life can feel meaningless to some people and the lack of friendships motivates us to meet people and fill the gap.

Esteem Needs
Everybody feels the urge to be independent, free, strong both physically and mentally and successful. As a passive part of our self-esteem we need the appreciation of other people.

Self-Actualization
When all other needs are satisfied, the need for self-actualization starts to wake up in us. It is the need to grow and develop and reach personal fulfillment.

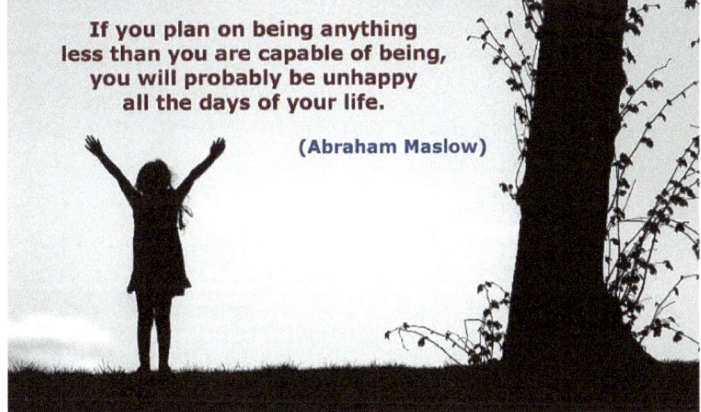

If you plan on being anything less than you are capable of being, you will probably be unhappy all the days of your life.

(Abraham Maslow)

Maslow believed that people would not move on down this list to be motivated by the next set of needs until the previous set(s) had been satisfied. For example, to somebody who has not enough food it is less important to be part of a social group than to find something to eat. Maslow was thus inspired to start a whole new movement in psychology – a third wave – which he called **humanistic psychology**.

This was a real departure from the two dominant theories of the time (Freudian human beings were almost entirely driven by primitive urges like sex and aggression / behaviorists' view, human beings are like oversized lab rats — programmed or *conditioned* to behave the way they do by factors outside of their control.) Humanistic psychology acknowledges a human or existential urge to grow, to seek happiness and fulfilment, to live up to our potential.

Unfortunately the western world seems to have stalled on social needs, and largely ignores the issues of esteem and self-actualization which are present in Teal organizations and the reason teal organizations enjoy such success. For Maslow, a high level of self-actualization reflects the fact that human beings are not simply biological machines. We are increasingly driven by a sense of personal meaning and purpose as we mature and become more aware of ourselves.

Many people are under the impression that the hierarchy of needs stops there. Not so.

For while studying people who operate at the level of self-actualization, Maslow noticed that many of them frequently have, and deliberately seek, some other kind of experience. He noticed something extraordinary.

Maslow termed these **peak experiences**. They are profound, life-altering moments of love, understanding, happiness, bliss. They are moments in which one feels radically more whole, more completely alive, more aware of truth, beauty, goodness, and so on.

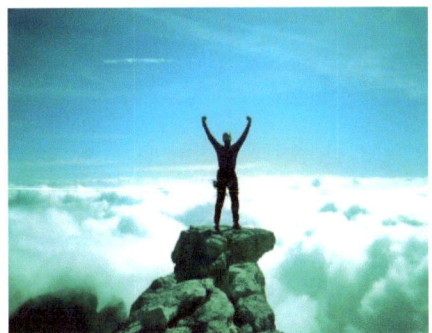

Self-actualizing people have many such peak experiences and eventually feel inspired to actively seek them, extend them and stabilize them. Hence, Maslow added the goal of **self-transcendence** as the final level, the capstone of the pyramid. The desire is to go beyond our ordinary human level of consciousness and experience oneness with the greater whole, the higher truth, whatever that may be.

The earliest and most widespread version of Maslow's hierarchy (based on Maslow's earlier work) shows only the first five levels. A more accurate version of the hierarchy, taking into account Maslow's later work and his private journal entries, shows six motivational levels, with self-transcendence at the top (Koltko-Rivera, 2006).

Alderfer's Theory

Clayton Alderfer developed a theory as an advancement of Maslow's Hierarchy of Needs in view of the needs of workers in a company. It distinguished those needs into three categories:

- Existence needs
- Relatedness needs
- Growth needs

Alderfer divided the human needs into basic and cultural needs. Basic needs include the need to eat, to drink and to reproduce. Also the urges of having a safe place and clothing and to be part of a social group are a basic part of human nature. Naturally, people also strive for power and leadership. All other needs a cultural dependent.

Once again, the theory here does not address the prime emotional information stream which is available to all people.

You can have growth, relate well, have a high level of safety, food and drink, yet feel like there is, as singer Robbie Williams says "*A hole in my soul, it's a real big hole*"

This is consistent with Maslow's motivation towards self-transcendence.
The issue with self-transcendence is that many people get stuck linking their perception of self-transcendence to religion. This is not valid if religion is a set of rules or beliefs imposed implicitly inherited or by force.

The modern profession of counselling is largely inspired by Maslow's "third wave", humanistic psychology.

The teal movement, which incorporates transpersonal psychology, inspired by peak experiences and the quest for self-transcendence, could constitute a "fourth wave" were it ever to become more accepted into the mainstream.

Most people seem to find Maslow's model of the hierarchy of needs intuitively satisfying. It makes a kind of sense — even though self-actualization is something many people have trouble relating to from personal experience.

Becoming "Teal" means to see live as a journey that leads to self-actualization. The goal is not being powerful or loved (that would the fourth need according to Maslow), but to discover who we really are. We cannot actively navigate to that point but we have to let go and see where living our lives brings us. Living in adventure takes us in search of our real purpose in life and service to our world.

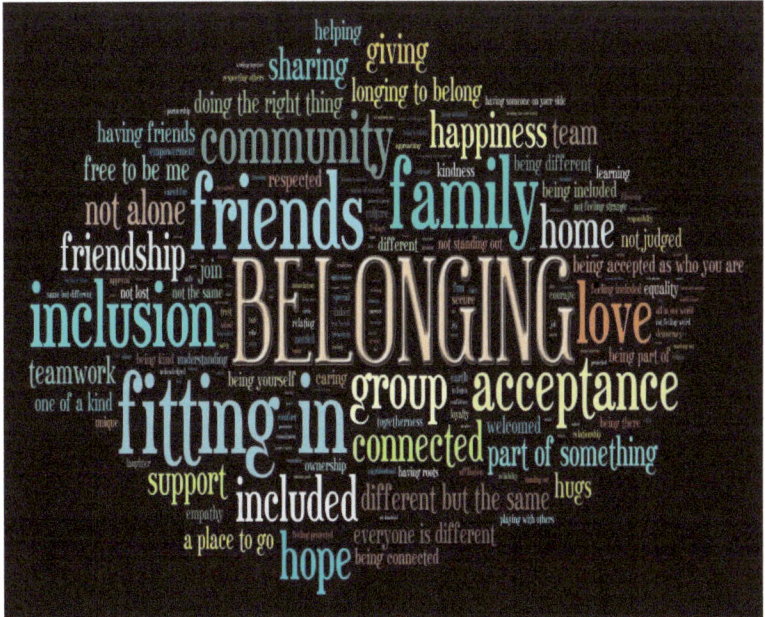

To what do we want to belong?
Do we desire only individualism, or limit ourselves just to our nuclear family? To the wider extended family? To those who believe in something we hold true (despite knowing that we can never define that something to everyone's agreement)? Or do we associate with a political or state boundary?

I suggest the human race is the highest form we can belong to, especially in its evolved form, which is described by these teal attributes:

Self-management within a wider community.

Respect the community, the source of wisdom in others, without having to submit or gain approval for your own ideas and thinking. This is critical, because most of us have been significantly hobbled by the views of others which are no longer serving us

Wholeness

Practice those virtues that invite and allow us to reclaim our inner wholeness, and to bring all of our passion and gifts to each day, instead of pasting ourselves into a corner defined by what others see us, our role in society, our work or our 'mojo'.

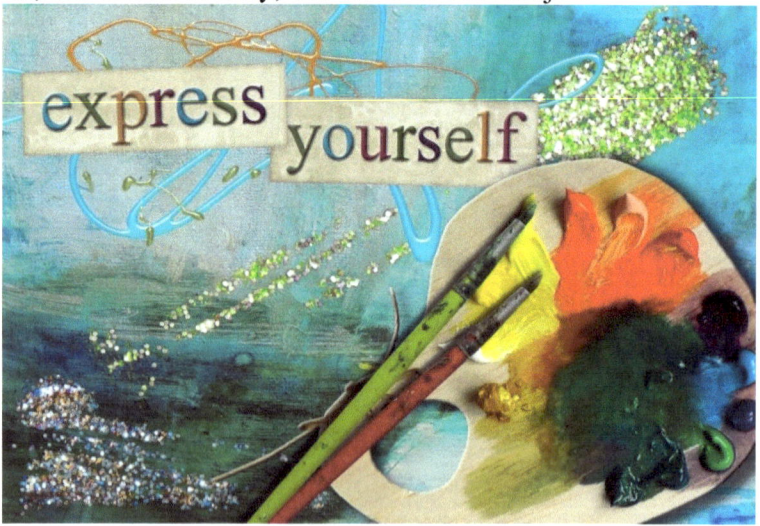

Evolutionary Purpose

Instead of trying to predict and control the future, start to listen and understand reality, from which clarity will emerge. We need to understand what our purpose is during this life, in order to fulfil it.

Working hard to climb a wall is ignorant, if conquering the wall leads you into a place you did not want to be in.

If each individual in a community has evolved to work in this way, then everyone wins in the workplace, too.

However bringing your individual awareness to seeing this as merely one part of a bigger picture will enable us to approach other community participation in the same way, including our spiritual community (Church/Mosque/Synagogue, etc.), our sports and hobbies, and most importantly, our families.
Imagine your family operating on these principles, with equal peer relationships, supporting each other's wholeness rather than seeking family conformity, and allowing each member of the family to contribute to a picture of what purpose it intends. Clarity at home is not utopian if the children are brought up with these principles.

Let's now look at these principles in more detail:

Trust
We should treat the people around as in a positive and friendly manner. If nothing proofs the opposite, it should be self-evident to trust every person in your life and always see the good inside people.

Information and decision-making
No information should be hold back from anyone. Even if we think we might protect people from being hurt we should always keep in the back of our head that everyone is able to handle all kind of news, also bad news. We should not put ourselves over others or consider us to be smarter than other people. For that reason we should not make decisions on our own but include everyone in the process of making decisions. With united intelligence we have the most power.

Responsibility and accountability

Every member of the community feels responsible for its positive development. We don't close our eyes to what happens around as and try to widen our horizon. Nobody should be afraid of committing themselves to the community.

Equal worth

All members of the society, all people on this world are of equal worth, nobody is better or worse than somebody else. Our community only profits from the diversity of its members. We should accept and appreciate the differences in race, gender, sexual orientation, education, religion, background, interest and so on.

Safe and caring community

In all our interaction with other humans it is important to create a safe space in which everyone can express themselves naturally. We should care for others and respect them.

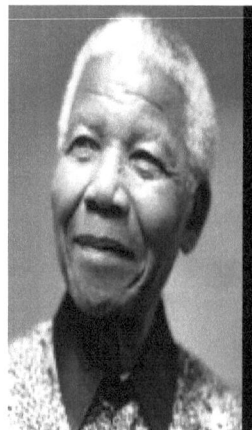

No one is born hating another person because of the colour of his skin, or his background, or his religion. People must learn to hate, and if they can learn to hate, they can be taught to love, for love comes more naturally to the human heart than its opposite.

(Nelson Mandela)

Overcoming separation

As we consider every people to be equal, we should work actively on overcoming separation in our society. A deeper connection unites all of us and we should fight for that.

Learning

Failure, mistakes and problems are a great opportunity to learn. We should reflect what went wrong and then learn from it. Remember that we will never stop learning our entire life and there will never be the moment when you suddenly know everything. Mistakes will only make us stronger. To support others in their learning process, we share respectful and fair criticism with them. Growing up we accept that losing is a natural part of life, and that we can never control another person's thought, and as we do so we open up to growth and learning.

Relationships and conflict

We can deal better with relationships to others if we always remember that we cannot change people, we can only change ourselves. To avoid conflicts we should not gossip and if it comes to an argument, we won't put uninvolved persons in the middle of it, but we solve it by our own. During an argument we should communicate positively, use I-statements and avoid generalizations. As we are responsible for what we belief, think and do, we should not blame our problems on others and never stop reflecting our behavior.

In the Western society, separation is everywhere, visible in all circumstances and very clearly in the work place. We behave different at work and at home and doing so, develop two different faces, a separation of ourselves that keeps us from "being whole".

Often the masculine, the rational, the ego is valued over the feminine, the emotional, the spiritual and sometimes these words are used in a negative context. Overcoming this separation is not easy because it's enrooted so deeply in people's minds. We need to live wholeness to realize that we are part of something bigger that connects us all with each other and in the same time we can express truly who we really are.

Given this new paradigm, there is considerable motivation to adapt to the latest stage of growth for personal satisfaction, corporate longevity, and sense of purpose, both short term, and for self-transcendence.

However don't think this is going hippie. The purpose of developing your own life-balance and putting that together with Jesus' golden rule of "Do unto others as you would have them do to you" is that way we work together can be transformed for the positive.

Collective purpose

When we start to see the organization or society as a living organism with a soul, we realize that it is connected to the same mysterious life force as us. It has its own purpose in life and we cannot force it to go in a special direction.

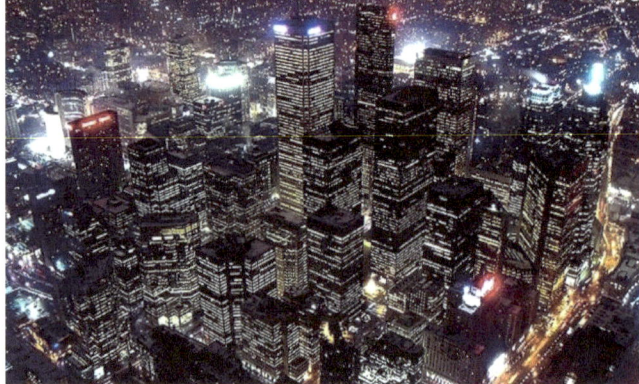

Individual purpose

The community is a part of our lives so have the same duties to it as we have to ourselves. We are a living part of it. We fulfill our roles in community without letting us getting ruled by our egos.

Planning the future

We cannot plan the future. Instead of trying to control it, we can let go and make decisions dependent on the current circumstances. We respond to what's happening right now, because we cannot influence the unpredictable. That's how we find the right way.

Profit

Reasonable acting leads to success. If we focus on purpose and with that find the right direction, profit and success will follow.

So it is with wholeness with life and nature.

If we continue our journey to find our true self, we will realize more and more that we are part of an interconnected web of life.

When we consider us as a part of nature, we will be able to fix our broken relationship with it. It will lead us to a simpler life and we will start to be aware of what we actually need.

We are not rich by things but by our relationship to nature.

Being part of the big thing will make us whole.

Practical tips to doing things consistent with your higher self

There are many approaches to reclaiming your true self. The main one is of course spending time getting to know who you truly are. But there are little steps too, that can be achieved while you struggle with the wider perspective from above.

If you want success, change a small habit or behavior.

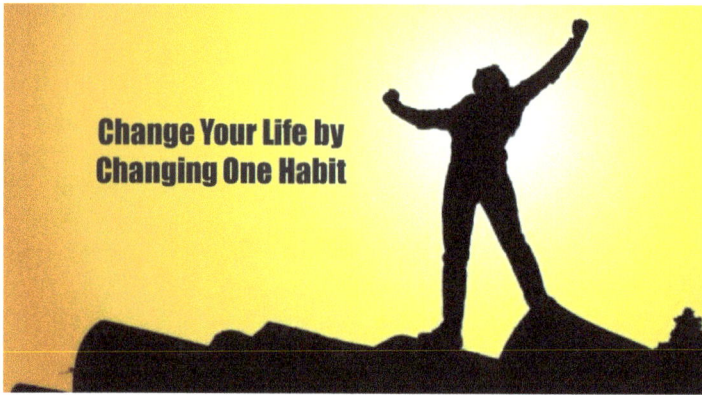

Not a big one, like quitting smoking. Something that you know you will succeed at now.

Incorporate a small routine, like writing things down.

Or try waking up 10 minutes earlier.

Drink a glass of water when you wake up. Something small that you know you can do.

Do it for a month. When you've achieved that, you'll feel like a million dollars. Here are some examples:

1. Groom yourself.

This seems like such an obvious one, but it's amazing how much of a difference a shower and a shave can make in your feelings of self-confidence and for your self-image. There have been days when I turned my mood around completely with this one little thing.

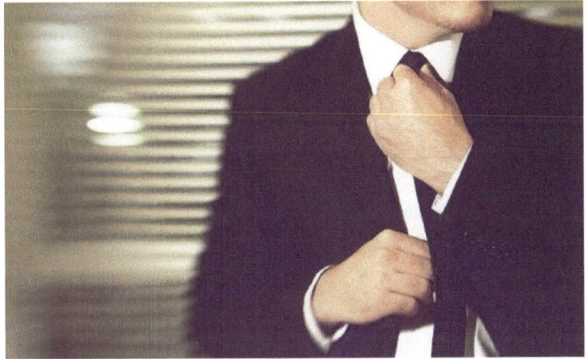

2. Dress nicely.

A corollary of the first item above … if you dress nicely, you'll feel good about yourself. You'll feel successful and presentable and ready to tackle the world. Now, dressing nicely means something different for everyone … it doesn't necessarily mean wearing a $500 outfit, but could mean casual clothes in which you're comfortable and that are nice looking and presentable.

3. Photoshop your self-image.

Our self-image means so much to us, more than we often realize. We have a mental picture of ourselves, and it determines how confident we are in ourselves. But this picture isn't fixed and immutable. You can change it. Use your mental Photoshop skills, and work on your self-image. If it's not a very good one, change it. Figure out why you see yourself that way, and find a way to fix it.

4. Think positive.

One of the things I learned when I started training for the Camino trail was how to replace negative thoughts (see next item) with positive ones. How I can actually change my thoughts, and by doing so make great things happened. With this tiny little skill, I was able to train for and run a marathon within a year. It sounds so trite, so 'Norman Vincent Peale', but it works. Seriously. Try it if you haven't.

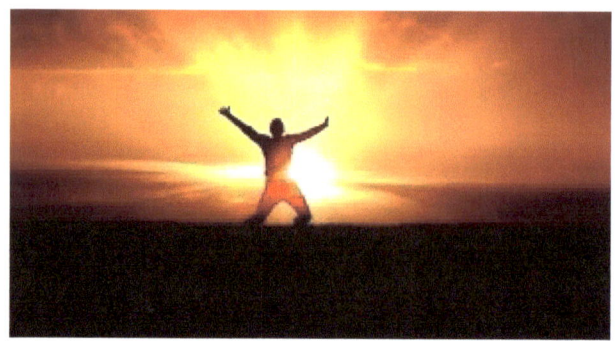

5. Kill negative thoughts.

Goes hand-in-hand with the above item, but it's so important that I made it a separate item. You have to learn to be aware of your self-talk, the thoughts you have about yourself and what you're doing. When I was running, sometimes my mind would start to say, "This is too hard. I want to stop and go watch TV."

I soon learned to recognize this negative self-talk, and soon I learned a trick that changed everything in my life: I would imagine that a negative thought was a bug, and I would vigilantly be on the lookout for these bugs. When I caught one, I would stomp on it (mentally of course) and squash it. Kill it dead. Then replace it with a positive one. ("C'mon, I can do this! Only one mile left!")

6. Get to know yourself.

"Know yourself and you will win all battles." – **Sun Tzu**

When going into battle, the wisest general learns to know his enemy very, very well. You can't defeat the enemy without knowing him. And when you're trying to overcome a negative self-image and replace it with self-confidence, your enemy is yourself.

Get to know yourself well. Start listening to your thoughts. Start writing a journal about yourself, and about the thoughts you have about yourself, and analyzing why you have such negative thoughts. And then think about the good things about yourself, the things you can do well, the things you like.

Start thinking about your limitations, and whether they're real limitations or just ones you've allowed to be placed there, artificially. Dig deep within yourself, and you'll come out (eventually) with even greater self-confidence.

7. Act positive.

More than just thinking positive, you have to put it into action. Action, actually, is the key to developing self-confidence. It's one thing to learn to think positive, but when you start acting on it, you change yourself, one action at a time.

You are not what you do, but if you change what you do, you change your perception of what you are. Act in a positive way; take action instead of telling yourself that you can't, be positive. Talk to people in a positive way, put energy into your actions.

You'll soon start to notice a difference.

8. Be kind and generous.

Oh, so basic. If this is too obvious for you, move on. But know that being kind to others, (generous with yourself, your time and your assets) is a tremendous way to improve your self-image.

You act in accordance with the Golden Rule, and you start to feel good about yourself, and to think that you are a good person. It does wonders for your self-confidence, believe me.

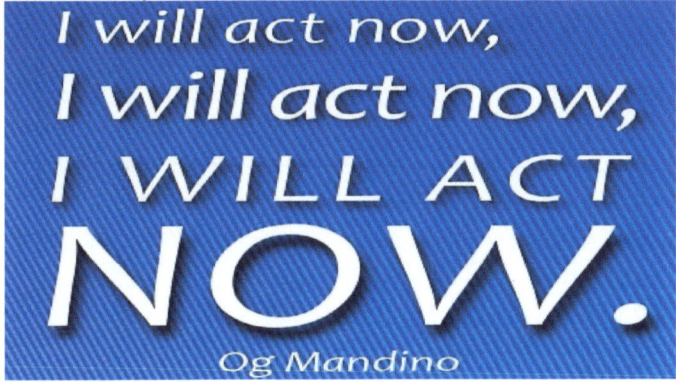

9. Get prepared.

"One important key to success is self-confidence. A key to self-confidence is preparation." – **Arthur Ashe**

It's hard to be confident in yourself if you don't think you'll do well at something. Beat that feeling by preparing yourself as much as possible. Think about taking an exam: if you haven't studied, you won't have much confidence in your abilities to do well on the exam. But if you studied your butt off, you're prepared, and you'll be much more confident.

Now think of life as your exam, and prepare yourself.

10. Know your principles and live them.

What are the principles upon which your life is built? If you don't know, you will have trouble, because your life will feel directionless. For myself, I *try* to live the "Golden Rule" (and fail often).

This is my key principle, and I try to live my life in accordance with it. I have others, but they are mostly in some way related to this rule (the major exception being to "Live my Passion"). Think about your principles … you might have them but perhaps you haven't given them much thought. Now think about whether you actually live these principles, or if you just believe in them but don't act on them.

11. Speak with confidence.

Such a simple thing, but it can have a big difference in how others perceive you. A person in authority, with authority, speaks without rushing. It shows confidence.

A person of low self-confidence will often speak quickly. That may be because he doesn't want to keep others waiting for something which is self-assessed as low value.

Even if you don't feel the confidence of someone who speaks slowly, try doing it a few times. It will make you feel more confident. Of course, don't take it to an extreme and make it super slow, but don't rush either.

Be confident about your voice. If speaking makes you feel uncomfortable, you can check in with a speech therapist, you might actually speak in a sound that's not your natural voice.

12. Stand tall.

I was once advised to stand tall when going for an interview. It works! When I remind myself to stand tall and straight, I feel better about myself. I imagine that a rope is pulling the top of my head toward the sky, and the rest of my body straightens accordingly.

You can ask a friend to feel that thread and pull it gently and you will feel how your whole body straighten up, giving you a better feeling of being present in the moment.

As an aside, people who stand tall and confident are more attractive. That's a good thing any day, in my book.

13. Increase competence.

How do you feel more competent? How do you become more competent?

By studying and practicing. Just do small bits at a time. If you want to be a more competent writer, for example, don't try to tackle the entire profession of writing all at once.

Just begin to write more. Try different types of writing; journal, diary, blog, write short stories, do some freelance writing. The more you write, the better you'll be. Set aside a specific number of minutes a day to write and the practice will increase your competence.

14. Set a small goal and achieve it.

People often make the mistake of shooting for the moon, and then when they fail, they get discouraged. Instead, shoot for something much more achievable.

Set a goal you *know* you can achieve, and then achieve it. You'll feel good about that. Now set another small goal and achieve that. The more you achieve small goals, the better you'll be at it, and the better you'll feel.

Soon you'll be setting bigger (but still achievable) goals and achieving those too. Coaching is about finding these goals within a client, which is the core objective of my practice as a Coach)

15. Focus on solutions.

If you are a complainer, or focus on problems, change your focus now.
Focusing on solutions instead of problems is one of the best things you can do for your confidence and your career. "I'm fat and lazy!"

So how can you solve that? "But I can't motivate myself!" So how can you solve that? "But I have no energy!" So what's the solution?

16. Play.

Einstein is quoted as saying,

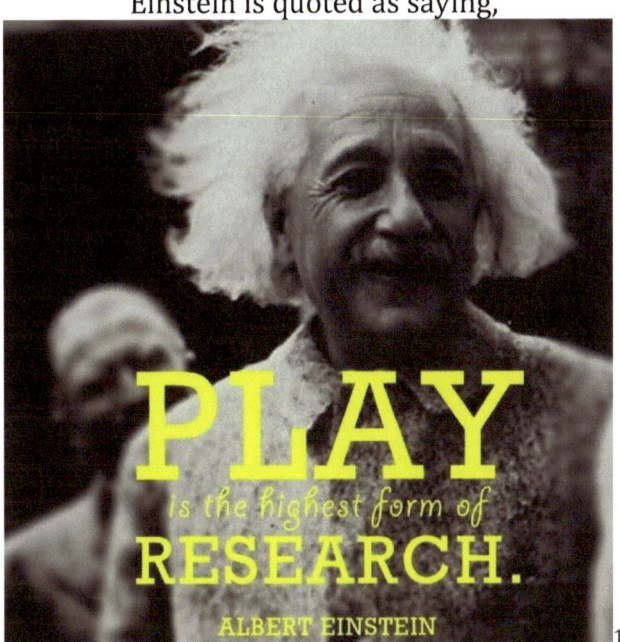

Play may be the best thing for finding out about ourselves, because we are letting go of logic. When did you last feel silly, and laugh crazily with others? Good, wasn't it?

I feel instantly better when I let go and laugh and it helps me to be kinder to others as well.

One little tiny act of fun can have a chain reaction. Not a bad investment of your time and energy.

---

[1] Einstein's actual quote was "The desire to arrive finally at logically connected concepts is the emotional basis of a vague play with basic ideas. This combinatory or associative play seems to be the essential feature in productive thought"

17. Volunteer.

Volunteering is related to the *"be kind and generous"* item above, but more specific. When it is the holiday season can you find the time to volunteer for a good cause, to spread some holiday cheer, to make the lives of others better?

It'll be some of the best time you've ever spent, and an amazing side benefit is that you'll feel better about yourself, instantly.

18. Be grateful.

I'm a firm believer in gratitude, as anyone who's been reading this blog for very long knows well.

I put it here because while being grateful for what you have in life, for what others have given you, is a very humbling activity … it can also be a very positive and rewarding activity that will improve your self-image.

19. Walk.

My wife and I walked the Camino Pilgrimage in Spain this year. 350 Kilometers. Today she showed me a quote that expressed the view that *the more you walk the more you know yourself.*

Exercise has been one of my most empowering activities in the last couple years, and it has made me feel so much better about myself. All you have to do is take a walk a few times a week, and you'll see benefits.

20. Empower yourself with knowledge.

Empowering yourself, in general, is one of the best strategies for building self-confidence. You can do that in many ways, but one of the surest ways to empower yourself is through knowledge.

This is along the same vein as building competence and getting prepared … by becoming more knowledgeable, you'll be more confident … and you become more knowledgeable by doing research and studying.

The Internet is a great tool, of course, but so are the people around you, people who have done what you want, books, magazines, and educational institutions.

22. Do something you've been procrastinating on.

What's on your to-do list that's been sitting there? Do it first thing in the morning, and get it out of the way. You'll feel great about yourself.

23. Get active.

Doing something is almost always better than not doing anything. Of course, doing something could lead to mistakes … but mistakes are a part of life.

It's how we learn. Without mistakes, we'd never get better. So don't worry about those.

Just do something. Get off your butt and get active — physically, or active by taking steps to accomplish something.

24. Work on small things.

Trying to take on a huge project or task can be overwhelming and daunting and intimidating for anyone, even the best of us. Instead, learn to break off small chunks and work in bursts.

Small little achievements make you feel good, and they add up to big achievements. Learn to work like this all the time, and soon you'll be a self-confident maniac.

25. Clear your desk.

This might seem like a small, simple thing (then again, for some of you it might not be so small). But it has always worked wonders for me.

If my desk starts to get messy, and the world around me is in chaos, clearing off my desk is my way of getting a little piece of my life under control. If you have any doubt about this read the book on Decluttering!

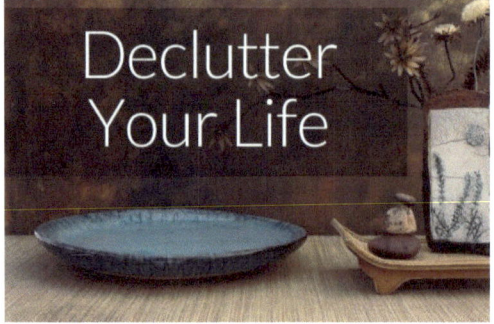

Energizing Work

So the bottom line of the issue of work life balance is that it is achieved by clarity of the connection between the two. If you are clear about being and doing, you will seek to achieve balance.

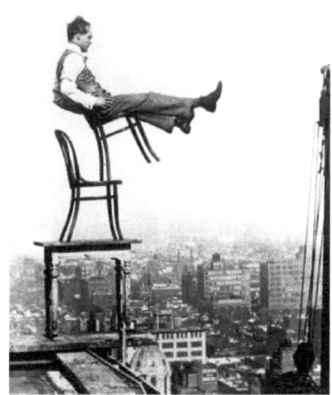

These are the yet unavailable energies you already have but now you will learn how to activate them and bring them to your organization:

You will feel more energized when you see a greater purpose in everything you do. When you work in an equal community without hierarchy you will find motivation and energy through self-management. When there's no boss anymore whom you have to follow without questioning, you will start to meet your inner standards which might be much higher, more demanding and therefor more motivation to work.

Of course, learning is always part of it, because it will always be a part of your life. You will not only improve your professional skills but also grow as a person.

A hidden talent is always a source of energy. It fulfills you when you can work with everything you got. When you are free of the boundaries of a limiting job, it opens up opportunities to use all of your talents.

In a Teal organization everybody is equal.

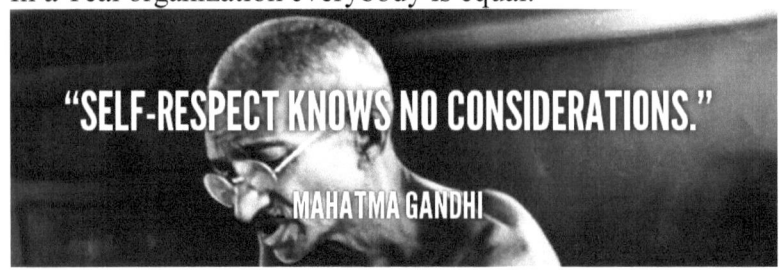

Respect for each other replaces the power struggle that comes with hierarchy. In Teal there is less wasted energy on the ego. Self-management also makes control mechanisms and useless meetings unnecessary.

These are the processes that took so much energy before Teal. Organizations can work with more energy, become more efficient as you discover energy sources that you may never have considered. The energy of the respected group holds not only great outcomes, but also a happier workday.

Practical tips to energize your work:

OK so now you have decided to change some behavior, what about the issue of energizing your work.

Let's be honest, most of us may want to move to higher ground in terms of loving our work, but those who are still stuck for the moment in a job that sucks, how can you take a small step forward in making that reality better?

Here is a list of ideas that may help:

1. Set your alarm 15 minutes earlier than you actually need to wake up, so you can rise gradually and mentally prepare for the day ahead. Always eat a healthy breakfast such as steel cut oats to kick-start your metabolism.

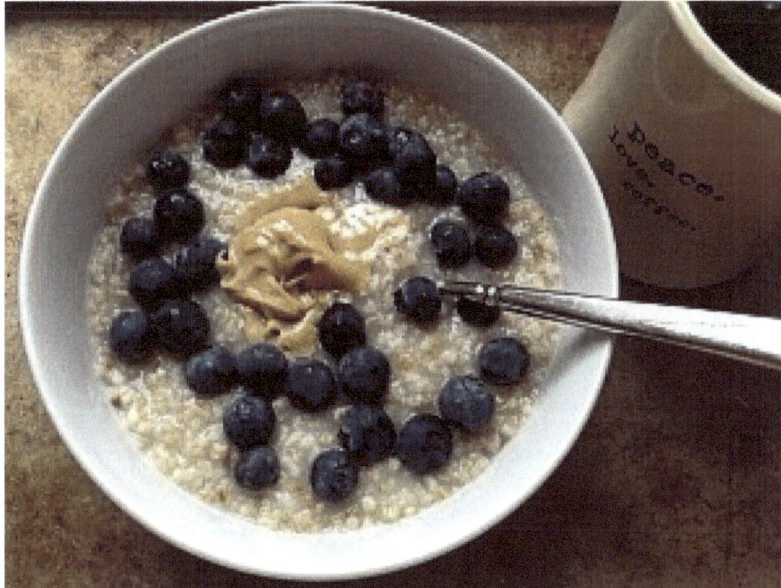

2. Researchers say commuting contributes to stress, exhaustion, and days missed from work. Aim to live close to the office.

3. A cluttered desk can cause stress, but it's not exactly easy to find the time to clean one up. The early morning, before tasks pile up and meetings come together, actually makes a great time to do so.

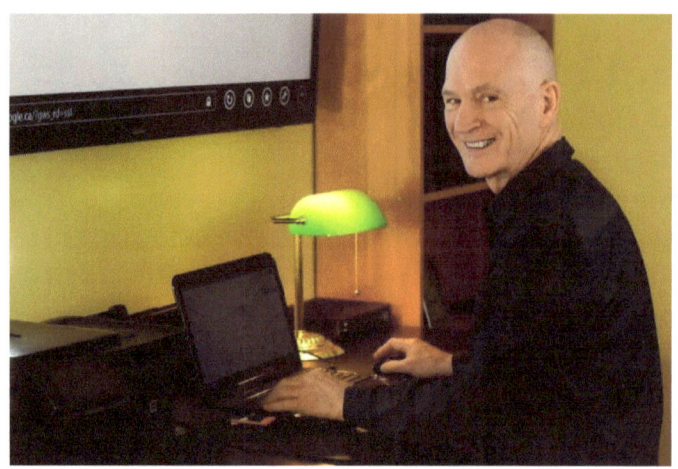

4. Too much coffee can lead to stress and even quirks in perception, so resist the urge to double down in one morning. If you've held out, 10 a.m. could be a good time to have a cup: since caffeine takes about 45 minutes to fully absorb, you'll be covered for a good chunk of the morning, and you won't have wasted any of your buzz before work's really underway.

5. Mid-morning munchies happen, but they may not do a whole lot to boost your energy level. Plus, a recent study suggests that they can obstruct weight loss. Eat away from your desk if at all possible to avoid a variety of health concerns, including serious bacteria. Nothing will sap energy like getting sick and staying in your chair all day.

    The prospect might sound a bit nutty, but consider this: Getting a little shuteye doesn't have to take much longer than a bathroom break or brewing a new pot of coffee. A mere 10 minute rest at 2 o'clock will boost your energy for the rest of the day. It's certainly worth a shot if you have a good spot available to you—try your car if there isn't vacancy in the office.

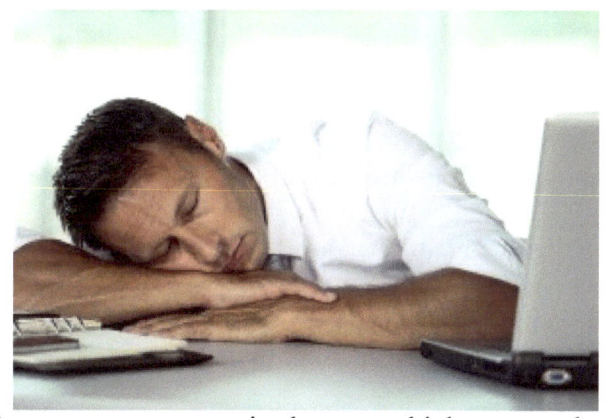

6.   Your eyes can get tired, too, which can make you feel bogged down. Try to stand up and take water breaks throughout the day to stay refreshed. Follow the 20-20-20 rule: Look at something 20 feet away from your monitor for 20 seconds every 20 minutes.

7.   There are several easy stretches you can do quickly at your desk, all of which can help you refocus on work. Many of which can be done without leaving your chair.

Try an exercise like the upper cervical spine flex every time you click "reply."

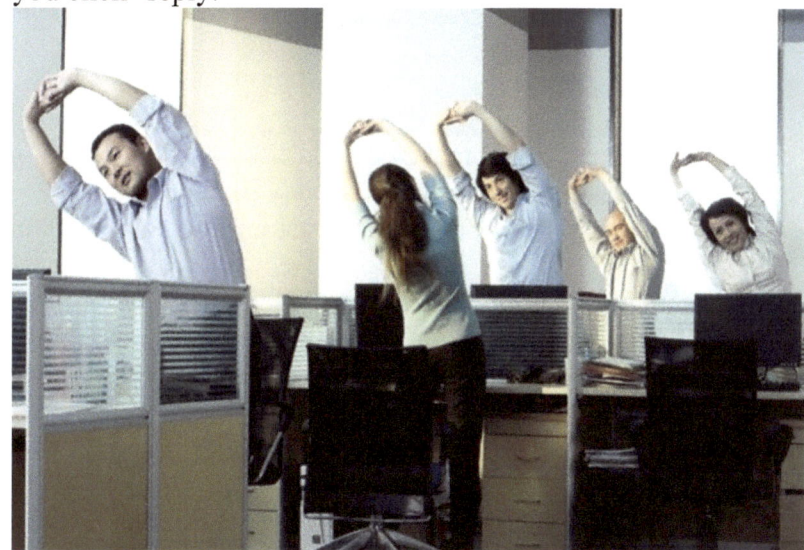

8. It's not always possible to leave right when the clock strikes 5—or 6, or whatever the end of your 8-hour workday might be—but try to get as close as possible. According to one study, working overtime can take a toll on your ticker, leading to serious health problems down the line.

   Don't rush out of the door. Instead, make sure you wind down properly: doing so will keep your energy up and spirits lifted as you head home. Have a chat with co-workers or watch a funny video before packing up.

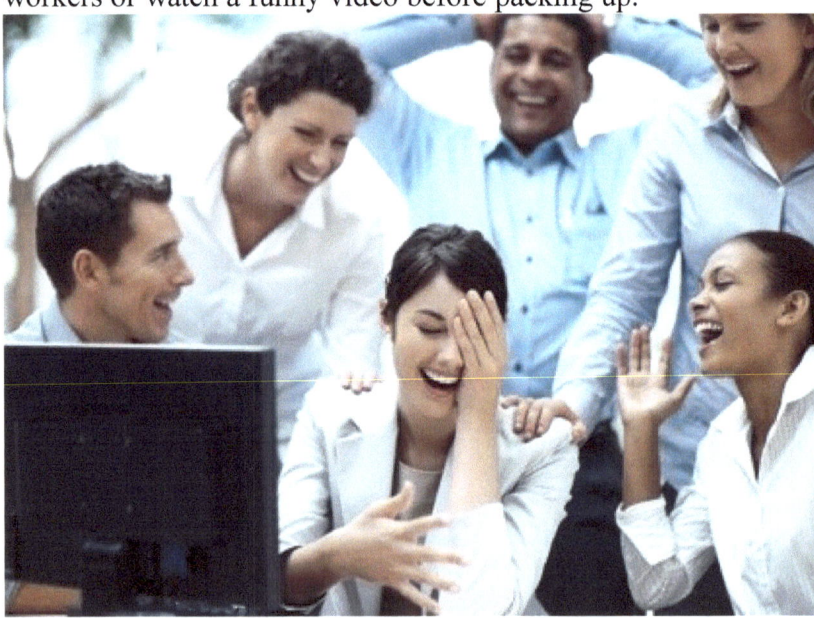

9. On the way home is a good time to rock out. If you're a music lover who's spent all day in relative silence, take the opportunity to pump up the volume a bit and unwind.

   It's just as important to practice mindfulness during your evening commute as it was in the morning—think of it as an opportunity to check back in with yourself and bring the day full circle. Plus, focusing on what's going on internally can help calm you down in the often stressful rush to get home.

10. To ensure another energized 9-5, you'll want to squeeze the most out of your nighttime shuteye.

There's more to it than shooting for eight hours of rest, though. Avoid bright screens—computers, smartphones, and TV—before you go to bed. Try a hot bath 30 minutes in advance, and keep a cup of water at your bedside: If you wake up feeling hot, lowering your body temperature will help you get back to sleep.

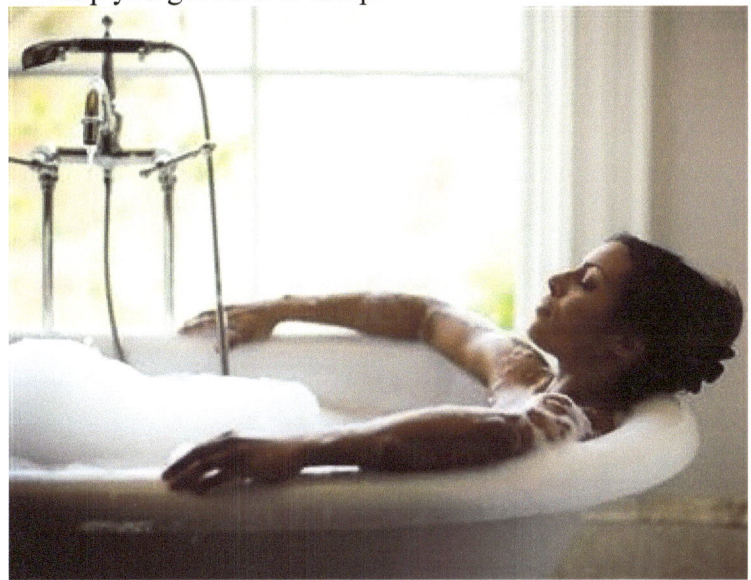

Work and life require each other.

When we stop separating between those two and see work as a part of our lives, we might feel more balanced.

Researchers like Frederick Laloux realized that as a logic development of humanity we need a shift to the next stage. When companies and organizations start to change their way of organizing to the Teal way, we as the workers will enjoy working more and our needs as humans will be met.

But also you need to reach the next stage. In which stage you see yourself? When you start to live after the Teal paradigm, you will start a journey that can lead you to who you really are and to a balance that you maybe never felt before.

Conclusion

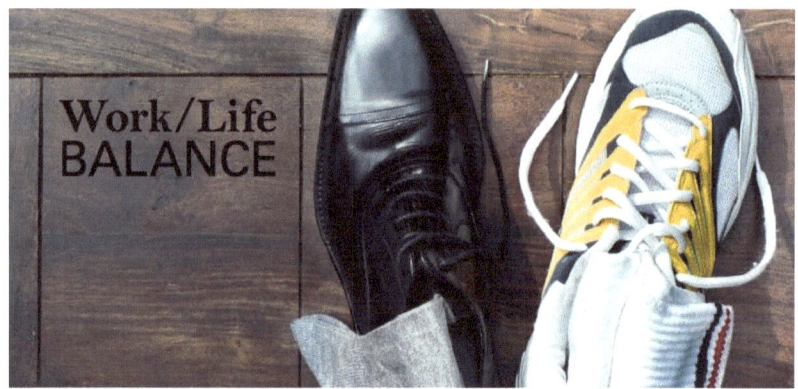

Energizing anything is to observer, to listen and to feel where the energy is. Strangely enough, connection to energy is not in the doing, or the roles, business, family, sport, art or mask that you wear.

Energy is always about being authentic to who you truly are, and therefore it has a spiritual aspect. It requires attending to the spirit within you that part of you that you do not understand, yet which seems to drive you.

Your spirit drives you to work, to play, to make decisions, yet we often deny it is the source of energy.

As Jim Rohn said in the opening quote to this book; "Success is neither magical nor mysterious. Success is the natural consequence of consistently applying the basic fundamentals."

The basic fundamentals are within you, and as a coach my role is to assist you in finding out the fundamentals of your passion, your drive, your bliss, and your spirit.

This is not magic, it is common sense. If your conscious mind is in tune with your subconscious spirit your life will glow with meaning, inspiration and creativity.

I welcome you to join me in experiencing this.

I really appreciate you reading this book!
Here are my **social media coordinates**:
Email me:

Phil@PhilCheney.com

Friend me on Facebook:

http://facebook.com/PhilosofreeCheney

Follow me on Twitter:

http://twitter.com/_Philosofree

Subscribe to my blogs:

http://www.philcheney.com/?page_id=10602 (Executive/ Life
Coaching)
http://www.diamondmine.me/blog (Abundant Life)

Connect on LinkedIn:

http://www.linkedin.com/in/Philosofree

Visit my Coaching website:

http://www.Advantace.com

Visit my Music & Art website:

http://www.DiamondMine.me

Author page

Amazon.com/author/philcheney

Other works by this author

Please visit amazon.com/author/philcheney or your favorite book
retailer to discover other books by Phil "Philosofree" Cheney.

Non-Fiction

Energizing Love: - a philosophy of holistic life

       Published by John Hunt Publishers, UK

Energizing Work: - the evolution of self towards authentic
balance in work and life (this book)

Fiction

The Bion& Freya Trilogy

Bion & Freya - Red Key - Asia & South America

Bion & Freya - Flight - North America & Europe

Bion & Freya - Scam - Africa & Australia

Poetry Series

Songs Above Notes - gratitude, humor and joy

Death of the Sun - renewal after suicide, grief and the loss of a
child (Available on request.)

Children's Book

Sambo Semo – Ages 3 to 8 year old – A simple tale about trust,
encouragement and having someone believe in you.
Beautifully illustrated in color by Carizza Los Baños